ANCIENT EGYPT Q&A

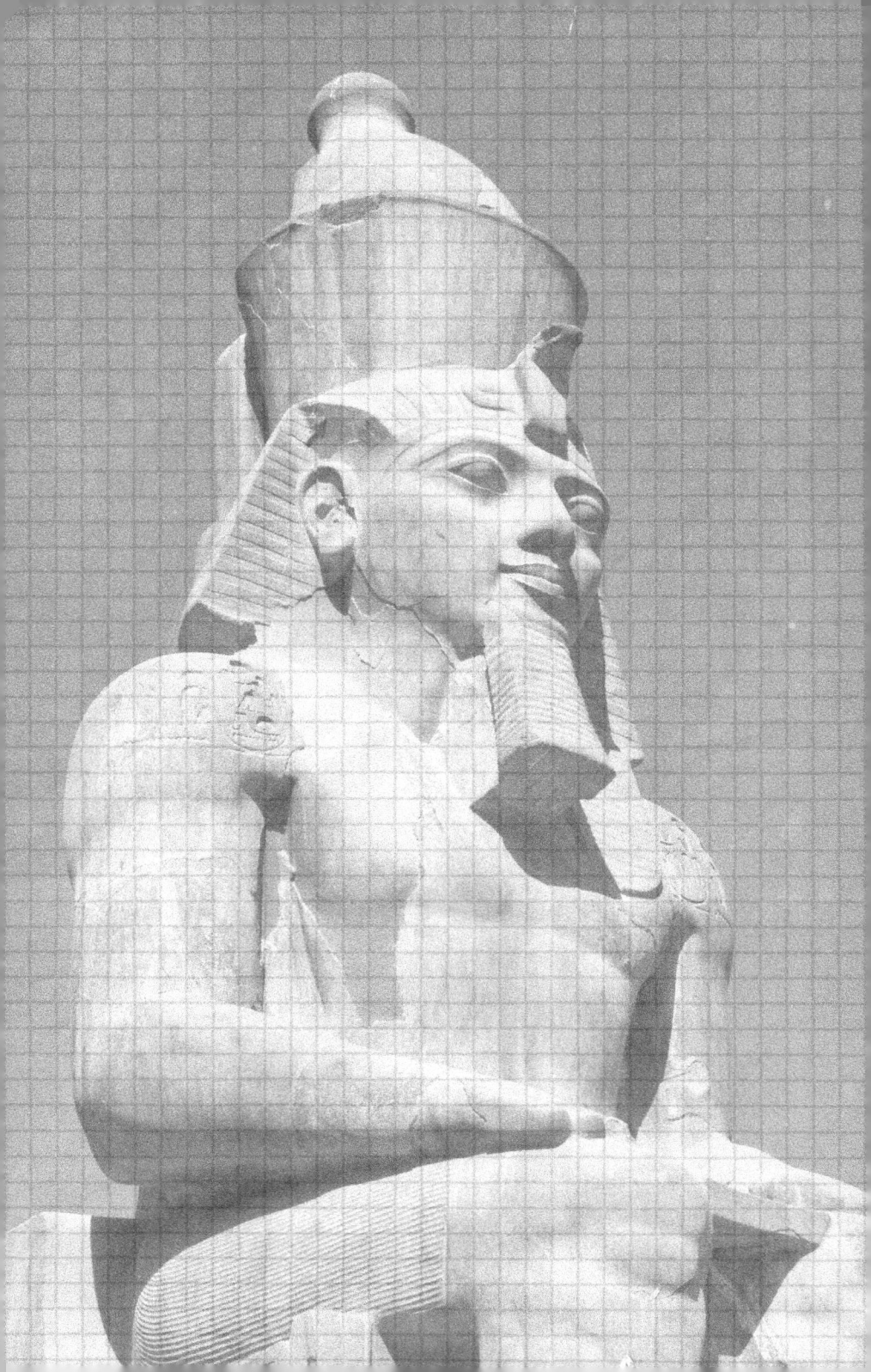

ANCIENT EGYPT
Q&A

175+ Fascinating Facts for Kids

CIARA O'NEAL

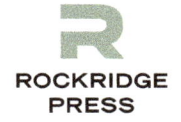

ROCKRIDGE PRESS

To my Lily, who inspires me to explore, adventure, and laugh.

Copyright © 2021 by Rockridge Press, Emeryville, California

No part of this publication may be reproduced, stored in a retrieval system, or transmitted in any form or by any means, electronic, mechanical, photocopying, recording, scanning, or otherwise, except as permitted under Sections 107 or 108 of the 1976 United States Copyright Act, without the prior written permission of the Publisher. Requests to the Publisher for permission should be addressed to the Permissions Department, Rockridge Press, 6005 Shellmound Street, Suite 175, Emeryville, CA 94608.

Limit of Liability/Disclaimer of Warranty: The Publisher and the author make no representations or warranties with respect to the accuracy or completeness of the contents of this work and specifically disclaim all warranties, including without limitation warranties of fitness for a particular purpose. No warranty may be created or extended by sales or promotional materials. The advice and strategies contained herein may not be suitable for every situation. This work is sold with the understanding that the Publisher is not engaged in rendering medical, legal, or other professional advice or services. If professional assistance is required, the services of a competent professional person should be sought. Neither the Publisher nor the author shall be liable for damages arising herefrom. The fact that an individual, organization, or website is referred to in this work as a citation and/or potential source of further information does not mean that the author or the Publisher endorses the information the individual, organization, or website may provide or recommendations they/it may make. Further, readers should be aware that websites listed in this work may have changed or disappeared between when this work was written and when it is read.

For general information on our other products and services or to obtain technical support, please contact our Customer Care Department within the United States at (866) 744-2665, or outside the United States at (510) 253-0500.

Rockridge Press publishes its books in a variety of electronic and print formats. Some content that appears in print may not be available in electronic books, and vice versa.

TRADEMARKS: Rockridge Press and the Rockridge Press logo are trademarks or registered trademarks of Callisto Media Inc. and/or its affiliates, in the United States and other countries, and may not be used without written permission. All other trademarks are the property of their respective owners. Rockridge Press is not associated with any product or vendor mentioned in this book.

Series Designer: Diana Haas
Interior and Cover Designer: Linda Kocur
Art Producer: Samantha Ulban
Editor: Eliza Kirby
Production Editor: Jenna Dutton
Production Manager: Martin Worthington

All images used under license © iStock and Shutterstock.

Paperback ISBN: 978-1-64876-792-0 | eBook ISBN: 978-1-63807-620-9
R0

INTRODUCTION

Desert sands. Grand pyramids. Mummified monarchs. Do these things have you picturing a certain place? You guessed it: ancient Egypt! But this civilization was so much more than that. Its people lived in a society filled with rich culture and mythology. Over the course of more than 3,000 years, ancient Egypt experienced times of great success, invention, and construction. Other times were filled with failure, famine, and war. Peasants, priests, and everyone in between celebrated life and the journey that came after death.

This book reveals the answers to all kinds of questions about ancient Egypt. Is there really a mummy's curse? Who actually built the pyramids? Did the Egyptians invent toothpaste? You're about to find out. As you go through the pages, you'll see trickier terms in **bold**. Use the glossary on page 73 to learn their definitions and uncover more about this fascinating culture.

Get ready to explore the wonders of ancient Egypt!

MORE THAN MUMMIES AND SAND

TRUE OR FALSE?

Egypt is a land completely covered in desert sands.

FALSE.

Although Egypt is mostly desert, the Nile River flows all the way through it. This river creates areas of rich, fertile land where plants grow.

Q **Where is Egypt located in Africa?**

A **Africa is a continent. It's made up of 54 countries. Egypt is just one of the countries in Africa. It is located in the northeastern area of the continent.**

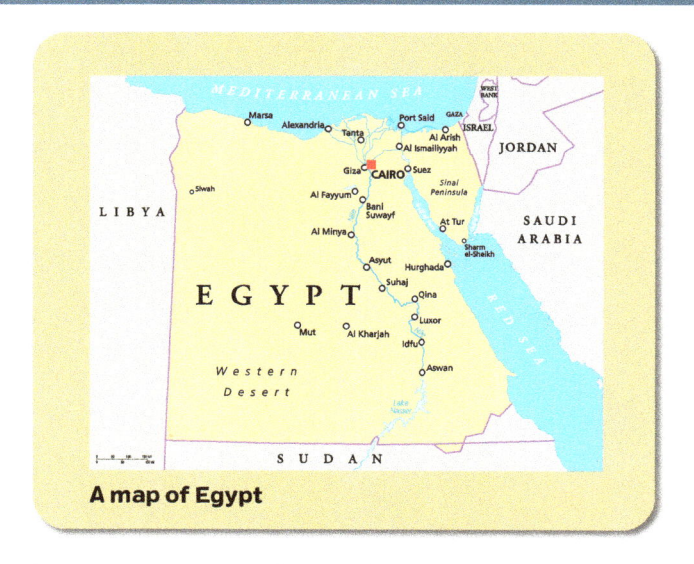

A map of Egypt

Q Was ancient Egypt isolated from the rest of the world because of its deserts?

A Harsh deserts, tall mountain ranges, and the Red Sea kept invaders out of Egypt. But that didn't mean the country was totally isolated. The Nile River made it easy for people to travel and trade goods by boat. Ancient Egyptians journeyed to distant lands and enjoyed visitors from all over Africa and Europe.

Stat: 95 percent of Egypt's population lived along the banks of the Nile. The other 5 percent were **nomads**, who moved from place to place.

Did You Know?

The Nile River surges and splashes over 4,100 miles. That distance makes it the longest river in the world.

Q Does the Nile split Egypt into two parts?

A Not really, no. The country does have two regions, though: Upper Egypt and Lower Egypt.

Myth:
Upper Egypt is north of Lower Egypt.

Truth:
Upper Egypt actually sits farther south. It's called Upper Egypt because it is uphill. Lower Egypt is located farther north, but is lower in elevation.

Stat: Only about 3 percent of Egypt's land is fertile enough to grow crops. Most of that land is located along the Nile River.

Myth:
The Nile River flows backward.

Truth:
The Nile *does* run from south to north, but the river is not magical, nor does it defy gravity. Its current runs that way because southern Egypt is on higher land and the water flows downhill.

Q How could the Nile River *flooding* be a good thing?

A For centuries, the Nile swelled from heavy rains during the annual wet season. The waters washed rich soil onto the banks. These floods allowed farmers to grow crops like wheat and flax.

Did You Know?

Ancient Egyptians built their homes on turtlebacks. No, not on real turtles. "Turtlebacks" are high pieces of land that became islands when the Nile's waters flooded the region.

Q Did the Nile's yearly flooding affect the Egyptian calendar?

A Yes! The ancient Egyptian calendar was divided into three main seasons: *Akhet*, the time of flooding, *Peret*, the growing season, and *Shemu*, the period for harvesting.

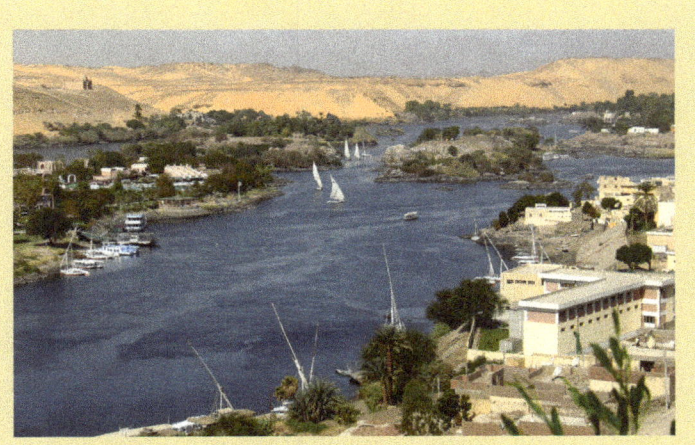

View of the Nile from the city of Aswan

Q What are the "gifts of the Nile"?

A Even though no wrapping paper was involved, the Nile provided many essentials that Egyptians considered gifts. It gave water, transportation, papyrus, soil for growing crops, and much more.

Q How did ancient Egyptians use papyrus?

A Papyrus was a plant that grew along the shore of the Nile. Egyptians used it for paper, but they also crafted many everyday items from it. The plant was used to make toys, clothes, medicine, and even boats.

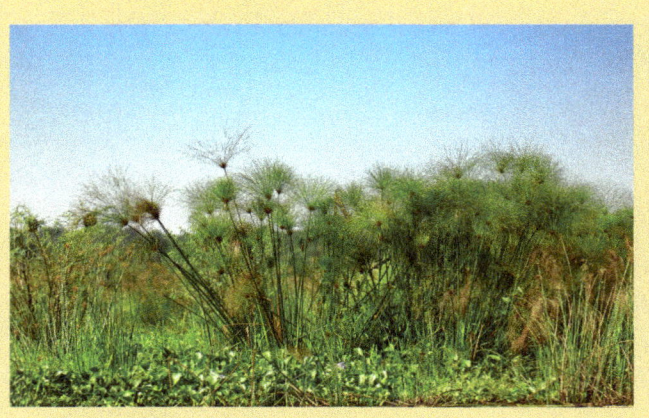

A papyrus plant on the Nile River

Did You Know?

Ancient Egyptians believed the god Amun-Ra pulled the sun across the sky in a boat made from papyrus reeds.

Q: Were the Nile waters safe for swimming?

A: No! Ancient Egyptians shared their land and water with some of the most aggressive animals on Earth, like hippopotamuses, crocodiles, jackals, and disease-carrying mosquitoes.

Did You Know?

Not many animals could survive the harsh desert climate. But the camel spider is one that can. These creatures were rumored to chase humans. In reality, they were just trying to cool off in people's shadows.

Myth:
Egyptian goods were transported from place to place by camels.

Truth:
Most Egyptian goods, like crops and cattle, weren't transported across the sandy dunes of the desert at all. Instead, the Nile acted as a watery highway. Goods were shipped by boat to markets and other cities throughout the ancient world.

Q Besides transporting goods, why were boats important to Egyptians?

A Boats were also used for worshipping the gods. They helped carry art from temple to temple and transported mummies to their final resting places.

TRUE OR FALSE?
The first Egyptian king, or pharaoh, was named "Catfish."

MOST LIKELY TRUE.
The first pharaoh was called Narmer. This name can be translated as "Fierce Catfish." Also known as Menes, he was the first ruler to unite Upper and Lower Egypt.

Did You Know?
Ancient Egypt's history is split into three major time periods. These eras are divided by where the kings were buried.

MAJOR TIME PERIODS OF ANCIENT EGYPT

TIME PERIOD	YEARS	WHERE WERE THE PHARAOHS BURIED?
Old Kingdom	2575 to 2130 BCE	**Pyramids:** Large stone monuments
Middle Kingdom	1938 to 1630 BCE	**Mastabas:** Rectangular rooms built into mountainsides or underground
New Kingdom	1539 to 1075 BCE	**Mausoleums:** Large underground burial rooms

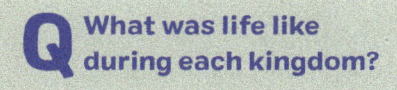

Q What was life like during each kingdom?

A Peace and prosperity filled the kingdom years. Strong governments led the people. The arts flourished. Monument building became fashionable among the pharaohs.

Q What were years like between the kingdoms?

A The years between the kingdoms were called the Intermediate Periods. These dark times were filled with plagues, famine, and quarreling kings.

Q How were each of the kingdoms different?

A The Old Kingdom saw growth in mathematics, art, and astronomy. During the Middle Kingdom, artistry of all kinds flourished. Egyptians made advances in literature, jewelry making, and other crafts. As for the New Kingdom, ancient Egypt was at the peak of its power. New lands were conquered, riches were reaped, and elaborate monuments celebrating the mighty pharaohs were built.

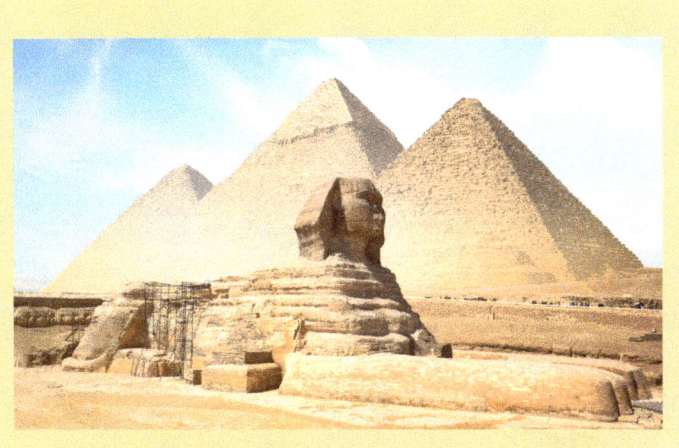

The Pyramids of Giza and the Sphinx

ANCIENT EGYPTIAN SOCIETY

Q: Could anyone become pharaoh?

A: No. Ancient Egyptians were born into social classes. These were generally determined by your parent's profession. If your father wasn't pharaoh, you had no hopes of becoming a king. Higher classes consisted of fewer people who enjoyed more power and wealth. Lower classes were made up of more people who didn't have the same privileges as the upper classes.

Myth:
Only men could be kings.

Truth:
Most pharaohs were male, but several women led ancient Egypt, including Hatshepsut and Cleopatra.

Did You Know?
Pharaohs were called king whether they were male or female.

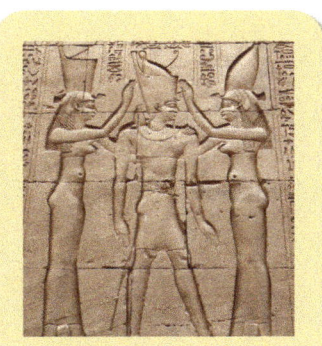

A wall carving at the Temple of Edfu showing a pharaoh

JOBS DETERMINED A PERSON'S RANK IN SOCIETY

JOB	DUTIES
Pharaoh	ruled the land and made laws
Advisor	helped run the government
Priest	served the gods, made mummies, cared for the temple gardens and statues, acted as doctors
Scribe	recorded all the daily data that affected Egyptian life
Soldier	fought wars, maintained weapons, policed the people, and even worked as farmers
Craftsperson, Merchant, or Artisan	created crafts, jewelry, woodworks, and delicious delicacies
Farmer	grew crops like barley, wheat, and vegetables
Servant or Enslaved Person	worked in mines, cleaned houses, plowed fields, and other duties

Q Did pharaohs rule Egypt all by themselves?

A The pharaohs of Ancient Egypt reigned **supreme.** But they never could have run the country alone. Instead, they relied on their **bureaucracy**. The officials who made up this class led armies, collected taxes, and advised the king.

Did You Know?

The chief judge and advisor to the king was called a **vizier**.

Q Besides making mummies, what did the priests do?

A Performing mummification was only part of their jobs. Priests also carried out rituals and ceremonies to worship the gods.

Myth:
All ancient Egyptians could read and write in hieroglyphics.

Truth:
Few Egyptians could read or write. It was the job of the scribes to record information for the nobility.

Stat: There are 26 letters in the English alphabet. The ancient Egyptian writing system has more than 700 hieroglyphs!

Q If people usually did whatever job their parents did, who could become a scribe?

A Anyone—even people from lower classes. However, becoming a scribe took a lot of time and money. Very few families could afford the school that lasted four or five years. A scribe's job involved complex duties, from counting the number of people in the country to helping determine the verdicts in court cases.

Did You Know?

When soldiers were not at war, they acted as police officers. These men were often second-born sons, since the eldest son inherited their father's lands and wealth.

Stat: Weapons, such as bows and arrows, were important to soldiers. Some warriors could hit a target from more than 600 feet away. That's almost the length of two football fields!

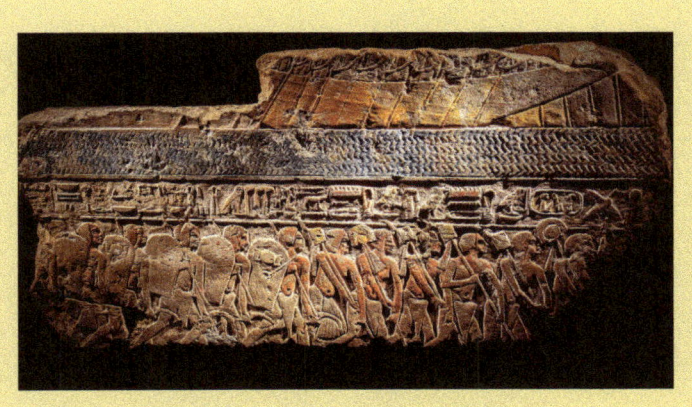

An engraving showing ancient Egyptian soldiers

Q Were artists and musicians rich and famous in ancient Egypt?

A No. Nobility, like the viziers and priests, lived in the lap of luxury. But craftspeople and artisans weren't well paid. Artists didn't even sign their names to their masterpieces. They were one of the lowest social classes—just above farmers, servants, and enslaved people.

Myth:
Ancient Egyptians paid for everything using gold.

Truth:
Ancient Egyptians didn't always use money. They **bartered** for the items they needed. For example, they might trade hay for fish or vegetables for clothing.

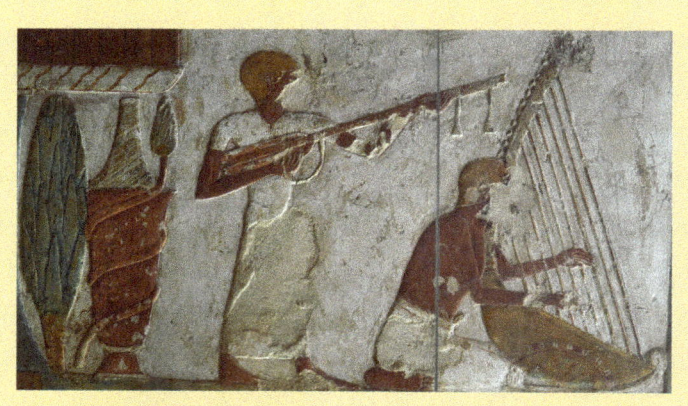

A wall painting showing Egyptian musicians

Stat: Farmers paid heavy taxes to the pharaoh—often up to 60 percent of their crops.

Stat: Up to 80 percent of the ancient Egyptian population were farmers, peasants, or enslaved people.

TRUE OR FALSE?

Enslaved people constructed the pyramids.

MOST LIKELY FALSE.

Popular culture and modern movies show men laboring under a burning sun while hauling heavy stones. There is no archaeological evidence proving this idea. Instead, evidence suggests that the pyramids were actually built by farmers who needed work when the fields were flooded. Historical finds even imply that they were fairly well paid.

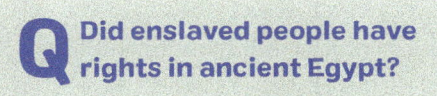

Q: Did enslaved people have rights in ancient Egypt?

A: Enslaved people were usually prisoners of war. In Egypt, they had more rights than most enslaved people throughout history. They could still own land, buy property, and marry whomever they wished.

Q How were Egyptian women treated differently from women in the rest of the ancient world?

A In ancient Egypt, women enjoyed much more freedom. They could inherit property, own land, bring lawsuits, serve on juries, and earn money. Some women even became pharaohs.

Did You Know?

Women wore linen dresses with detachable sleeves. They could remove this part of their outfit if they grew too hot. Dressing this way helped combat the heat of the desert.

Q Were appearances important to ancient Egyptians?

A Very! Men and women alike focused on their appearance and hygiene. Aside from bathing every day in order to keep fresh, wealthier Egyptian men and women wore makeup, jewelry, and fashionable clothing.

WHAT DID EGYPTIANS TYPICALLY EAT?

TYPE OF FOOD	EXAMPLES
Vegetables	lentils, lettuce, cabbage, beans
Grains	wheat, barley, flax
Fruit	dates, figs
Meats	goat, fish, pig, sheep, cow

Myth:
Children were not allowed to drink beer in ancient Egypt.

Truth:
People of all ages drank a goopy beer made from barley.

Did You Know?
Men held mock wars on the water where they attempted to knock each other off rafts.

Q What did Egyptians do for fun?

A Egyptians enjoyed many activities like sports (such as floor hockey and tug-of-war), board games (such as Senet and Twenty Squares), and festivals.

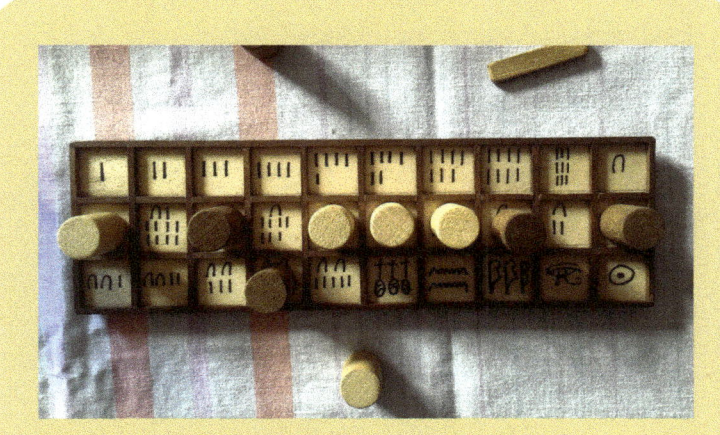

Egyptians loved games of all kinds, especially board games.

ANCIENT EGYPTIAN SOCIETY

MIGHTY RULERS OF EGYPT

Stat: There were 30 **dynasties**, or ruling families, that reigned over ancient Egypt for 5,000 years.

Q Why do historians disagree about who ruled and when?

A There isn't a complete list of the succession of Egyptian kings. Most records are incomplete or damaged. Archaeologists combine several sources to piece together history. These sources include a papyrus scroll called the Turin Canon and the Abydos King List, which is carved onto the stone walls of the Abydos temple.

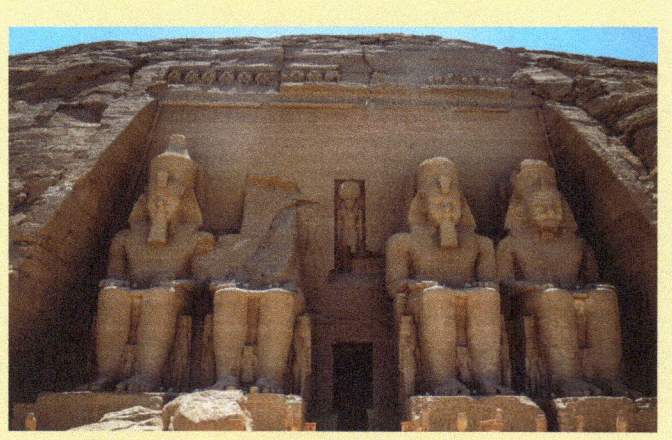

Statues of famous pharaohs

Q Did the Egyptians always call their kings "pharaoh"?

A Nope. The word "pharaoh" did not originally mean king. It meant "great house," or palace where the Egyptian kings lived. Only later did the people adopt this word as a sign of respect for their king.

Myth:
Pharaohs always wore beards.

Truth:
Most ancient Egyptians were clean shaven, but pharaohs were depicted in artwork with long beards. Beards were considered divine, so pharaohs wore fake metal beards to be godly—even the women!

Q How were pharaohs different from modern-day presidents?

A Like today's presidents, they ruled the people by creating laws, distributing resources, and commanding the armies. Unlike today's presidents, pharaohs were not elected. They were supreme rulers who acted as the link between humanity and the gods.

Did You Know?

Ancient Egyptians believed that pharaohs were the god Horus dwelling in a human body.

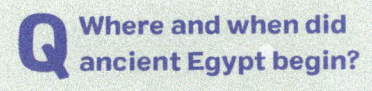

Q: Where and when did ancient Egypt begin?

A: The reign of the first pharaoh, King Menes, is considered the beginning of the first ancient Egyptian dynasty. His reign started about 3100 BCE. Menes's capital city was White Wall, later called Memphis.

Did You Know?

Pharaohs' wives were the second most powerful people in the land.

Stat: During the Old Kingdom, pharaohs divided Egypt into 42 territories called "nomes."

TRUE OR FALSE?

The head of a nome was known as a nomarch.

TRUE.

Nomarchs were governors appointed by pharaohs to rule the people and land.

Q What was a day in the life of a pharaoh like?

A Pharaohs had busy days filled with different people. Servants bathed and dressed them. Ambassadors visited them. The pharaoh collaborated with priests to perform rituals that kept Egypt safe. Bodyguards accompanied the pharaoh wherever they went.

Q What were those objects that the pharaohs always seemed to be holding?

A Pharaohs held a crook and a flail. These objects were symbols of kingship. The crook represented the pharaoh's role as the shepherd of their people. The flail was a stick-like weapon that shepherds used to defend their flock.

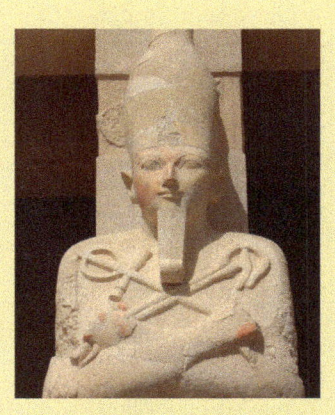

Statue of Queen Hatshepsut holding a crook and flail

MIGHTY RULERS OF EGYPT

Q Why do pharaohs wear snakes on their heads?

A Pharaohs did not use snakes for hats. They are often depicted with cobras riding their brows in Egyptian art. Cobras were a symbol of protection and were thought to ward off enemy attacks, usually by spitting flames at pharaohs' enemies.

Did You Know?

Pharaohs were said to have images of bound captives from enemy nations drawn on the soles of their shoes. So, whenever they walked, they crushed their enemies under their feet.

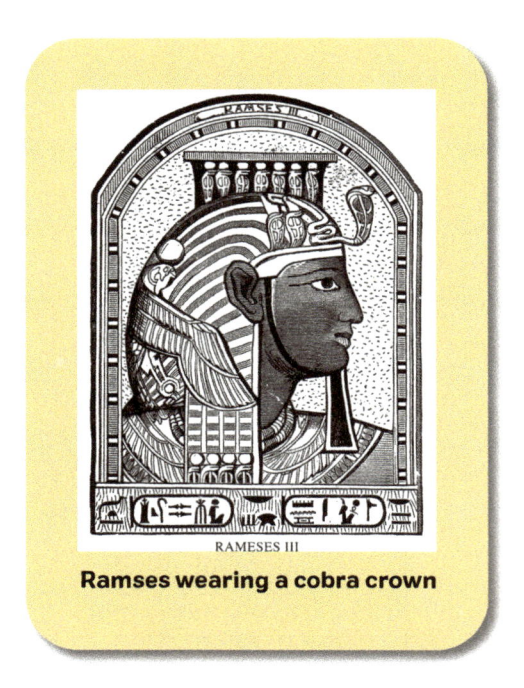

RAMESES III

Ramses wearing a cobra crown

24   ANCIENT EGYPT Q&A

Did You Know?

The Age of Pyramids began when the pharaoh Djoser asked the first known vizier, Imhotep, to build him the Step Pyramid.

Q Not much is known about pharaoh Khufu. Why was he important?

A Khufu is believed to be one of the first Egyptian kings to establish themselves as both a political and religious leader. He also declared that his afterlife temple should be filled with all the luxuries he had experienced when he was alive.

Stat: Khufu built the Great Pyramid of Giza as his **tomb**. It was the tallest structure in the world for more than 4,000 years.

Stat: The Great Pyramid of Giza took more than 2 million blocks and 20 years to complete.

TRUE OR FALSE?

Ancient Egyptians kissed the feet of the pharaohs.

TRUE.

Egyptian kings were believed to be living gods. Citizens lucky enough to meet the pharaoh considered it an honor to kiss the legs and feet of their leader.

Q Sons usually inherited the role of pharaoh from their fathers. How did Hatshepsut become the first female pharaoh?

A Hatshepsut's husband, Thutmose II, died when his son was two. Hatshepsut became Thutmose III's regent. Later, she appointed herself the first female pharaoh. She ruled for 22 years before disappearing from Egyptian records.

Stat: The entrance to Hatshepsut's tomb was guarded by at least six colossal sphinxes.

Q How did pharaohs' jobs change as Egypt grew?

A During the New Kingdom, Egypt conquered many of its neighbors. Egyptian kings became "warrior pharaohs" who fought alongside their soldiers.

Q Why is Thutmose III considered one of the greatest pharaohs of all time?

A After taking over from Hatshepsut, Thutmose proved himself to be a mighty king. He conquered Syria, defeated the kingdom of Mitanni, and conquered Nubia to the south. During his reign, Egypt reached the peak of its power and wealth. Many monuments and temples were built displaying his daring deeds.

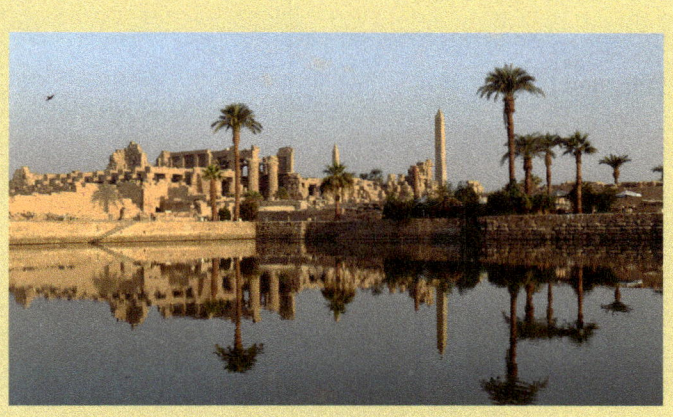

Thutmose III expanded the temple at Karnak.

Myth:
Most of the statues erected by Egyptians have fallen or been destroyed.

Truth:
Time has taken its toll on the statues, but many monuments remain. Amenhotep III, the grandson of Thutmose III, has the most statues left. There are more than 250 still standing!

Q Why did Egypt prosper under the rule of Amenhotep III?

A Amenhotep came into power at the age of 12. Fortunately for him, his father left him a powerful and wealthy kingdom. Amenhotep became a great ruler by forming **alliances** with other countries and keeping a tight grip on his people and priesthood. He had many new temples and monuments constructed.

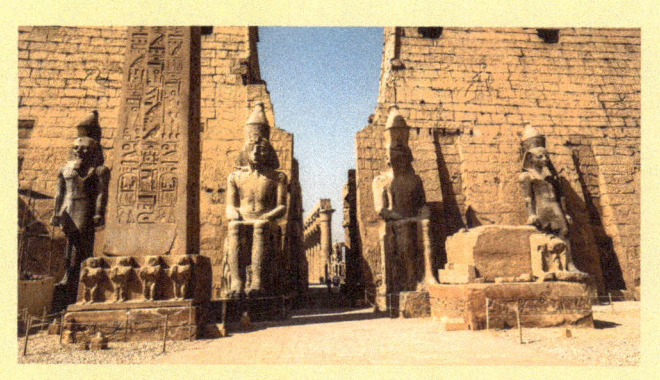

The entrance of Amenhotep III's temple at Luxor

Did You Know?

Egyptians were **polytheistic**, which means they worshipped many different gods. Their main god was Amun-Ra.

Q Why was the pharaoh Akhenaten known as the heretic king?

A Akhenaten wanted his people to worship one god: Aten. He changed his name from Amenhotep IV to show his devotion to Aten. Akhenaten even went so far as to move Egypt's capital from Thebes to a new city called Akhetetaon. The people and the priests were not pleased with these changes. Egyptian society returned to the old ways not long after Akhenaten's death.

TRUE OR FALSE?

Ancient Egyptians did not have a word for "queen."

TRUE.

In place of the word "queen," Egyptians used phrases like "King's Great Wife" or "King's Mother."

Myth:
Nefertiti was a pharaoh.

Truth:
Nefertiti ruled alongside her husband, Akhenaten. Although she was very powerful and held the title "God's Wife," she never became a king.

Q Why is Tutankhamun known as the "boy king"?

A King Tut inherited the throne when he was around nine years old. He reigned about 10 years before he died. His tomb was discovered in 1922 CE. The discovery of his burial site is one the greatest historical findings in the last century.

TRUE OR FALSE?

King Tut's original name wasn't Tutankhamun.

TRUE.

The boy king was born Tutankhaten. When he became pharaoh, he wanted to bring Egypt back to the old ways of worship that centered on the god Amun, so he changed his name.

Did You Know?

Tutankhamun was buried with his favorite board game. Egyptian royalty filled their tombs with all the necessary things for a luxurious afterlife like food, games, and even mummified animals.

> **Stat:** Tut's tomb was filled with more than 5,000 treasures to keep him entertained in the afterlife.

Q Who led the Egyptian army in the largest chariot battle in history?

A Ramses II. Both a military genius and brave warrior, Ramses led the charge against the invading Hittite army. Between 5,000 and 6,000 chariots fought at the city of Kadesh in Syria. The battle didn't go well for the Egyptians. Ramses II barely escaped with his life. But he survived and went on to become one of the greatest pharaohs in Egyptian history.

Did You Know?

Despite having many skirmishes with other countries, Ramses II signed the first international peace treaty.

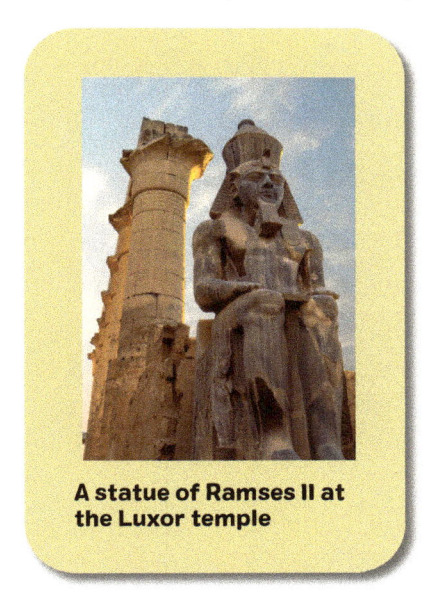

A statue of Ramses II at the Luxor temple

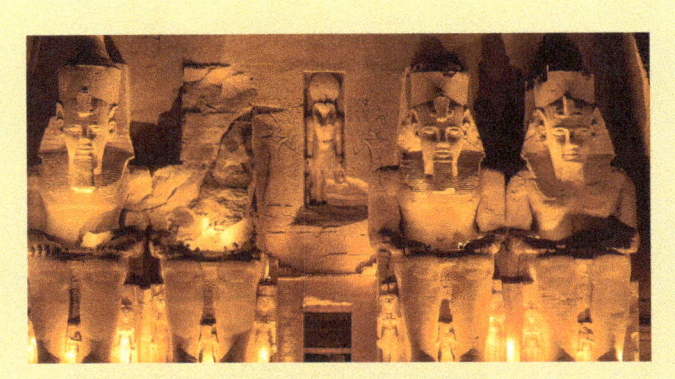

The entrance to the Great Temple of Ramses II

NUMEROUS NUMBERS ABOUT RAMSES II

- **became prince** regent at age 14
- **officially took** the throne at age 25
- **reigned for** 66 years
- **married more** than 200 wives
- **fathered more** than 100 children
- **was succeeded** by his 13th son

Did You Know?

Ramses II's reign was the second longest in Ancient Egypt. King Pepi II holds the record with his reign of more than 90 years.

TRUE OR FALSE?

The last true pharaoh of ancient Egypt was male.

FALSE.

Cleopatra VII, a female pharaoh, was the last king to rule Egypt.

Did You Know?

Cleopatra assumed the throne at age 18. She shared it with her 10-year-old brother, Ptolemy XIII.

CLEOPATRA'S ROCKY REIGN

69 BCE: Cleopatra VII is born.

51 BCE: She becomes pharaoh, but is driven into **exile** not long after by her brother.

47 BCE: Cleopatra regains the throne after defeating her brother with the help of Roman leader Julius Caesar.

44 BCE: Julius Caesar is murdered.

42 BCE: The Roman general Mark Antony meets and falls in love with Cleopatra.

37 to 32 BCE: Egypt works reluctantly with the Roman emperor, Octavian.

32 BCE: Octavian declares war on Egypt.

31 BCE: Octavian defeats Cleopatra's army at the Battle of Actium.

30 BCE: Cleopatra allows a snake to bite her and dies. Egypt becomes part of the Roman Empire.

RELIGIOUS ROLES

Did You Know?

Ancient Egyptians used religion to explain every aspect of their lives from mysterious **phenomena** in nature to life after death.

Q Whose job was it to keep the gods happy?

A First and foremost, that job belonged to the pharaoh. It was important to take good care of the gods and goddesses. The deities balanced *ma'at*: harmony, truth, and order. If the gods weren't pleased, they might not protect Egypt from the darkness and chaos that lurked in the land.

Myth:
Pyramids were places of worship for Egyptians.

Truth:
Temples, not pyramids, were the earthly homes of the deities. Most temples were the heart of a city. People gathered there to work, socialize, and bring offerings to statues of the gods.

Stat: The temple of Karnak is the largest Egyptian temple. It sits on more than 200 acres and is more than 2,000 years old.

Q Who cared for the temples?

A Priests were in charge of temples and all the activities that went on there. They didn't actually preach or hold religious services. Their role was to care for the deities. Only they could enter the inner parts of the temple.

Did You Know?

Egyptians believed that gods temporarily **dwelled** inside statues. So, the **clergy** set out food, washed and dressed statues, and even sprinkled them with perfume!

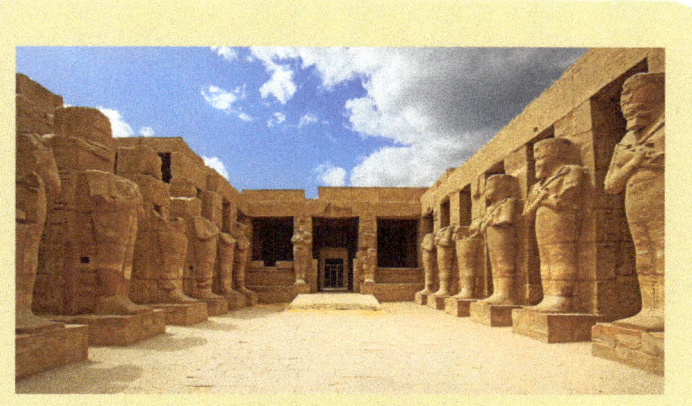

Giant columns at the Temple of Karnak

Q How did Egyptians worship their gods?

A Everyone from farmer to pharaoh attended religious festivals held by the priests. However, worshipping a god mostly took place in private. The Egyptian people mainly worshipped by giving gifts at personal shrines.

Q Were priests only male?

A No. Both men and women could be priests. Women usually served female gods and men served male gods.

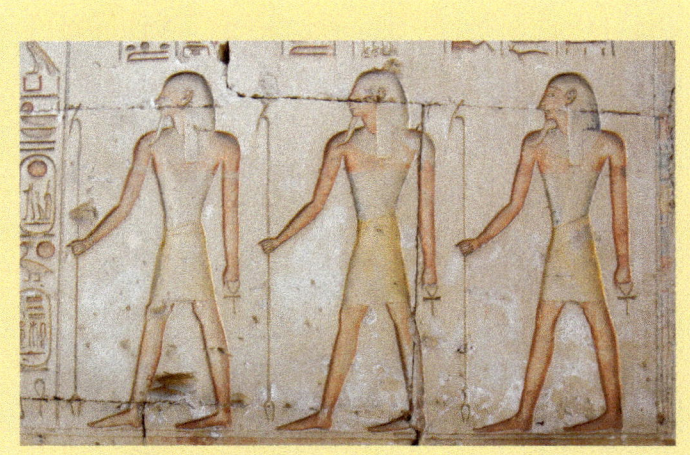

Three Egyptian priests

TRUE OR FALSE?

Ancient Egyptians believed that gods and goddesses took animal forms.

TRUE.

Egyptian art often depicts deities as having human bodies with animal heads.

SACRED ANIMALS IN ANCIENT EGYPT

ANIMAL	ASSOCIATED WITH THE GOD OR GODDESS	SYMBOLISM
ram	Amun	fertility
dog	Osiris	death and the afterlife
hawk	Horus	the sky and protection
cat	Bastet	grace and protection from illness
jackal	Anubis	judgment after death
ibis/baboon	Thoth	art and writing
scarab beetle	Ra	rebirth of the sun

TRUE OR FALSE?

Ancient Egyptians feared and hated crocodiles.

FALSE.

Egyptians had a healthy respect for the scaly beasts. They also worshipped the crocodile god, Sobek. It's said the waters of the Nile rose from his sweat!

RELIGIOUS ROLES

Myth:
Only cats were kept as pets in Ancient Egypt.

Truth:
Exotic animals displayed power and wealth, so creatures like baboons, monkeys, and gazelles were kept as pets, too. But Egyptians also kept more domestic creatures like cats and dogs.

Did You Know?

Only one god had the power to transform themselves into a cat: Bastet. She protected the people from disease.

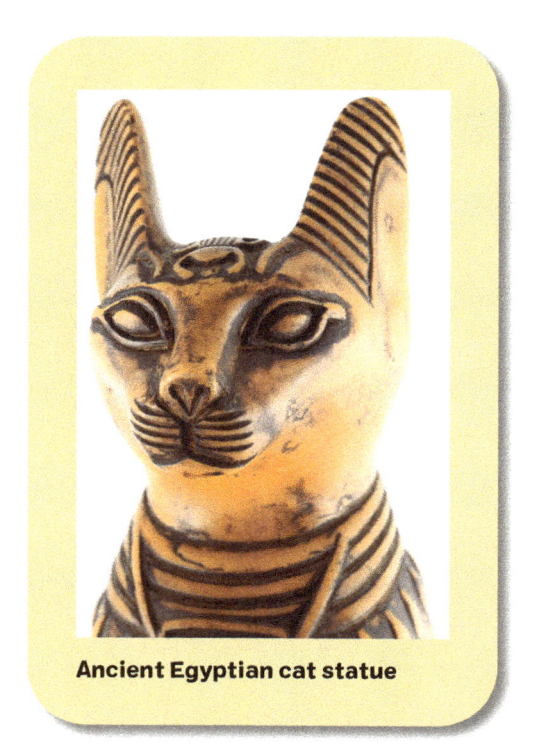

Ancient Egyptian cat statue

Q: Did Egyptians worship cats?

A: Egyptians did not worship cats, but these animals held a special place in the Egyptian heart. To honor their feline friends, Egyptians dressed them in jewels and fed them delicacies. It was even against the law to kill a cat. To do so was punishable by death!

Did You Know?

When a cat died, its owner would mummify its body. As a sign of grief, the owner would also shave their own eyebrows.

TRUE OR FALSE?

Animals were mummified to keep their owners company in the next life.

FALSE.

Pets were mummified, but it was about much more than friendship in the afterlife. The animals were gifts to the gods to help buy goodwill and favors.

TRUE OR FALSE?

Egyptians believed that gods and goddesses represented parts of nature.

TRUE.

Each Egyptian god explained a different phenomenon in the world. For example, the sun god, Ra, embarked on a daily journey that created day and night.

Did You Know?

Egyptians believed that humans sprang from Ra's tears. After seeing the world was a perfect and happy place, Ra began to cry and this created humans.

Q: Who exactly was the king of the ancient Egyptian gods: Ra or Amun?

A: It depends. At the beginning of ancient Egyptian history, Ra alone was the chief god. Over time, he was combined with the god of the sky, Amun. When Ra was combined with Amun, he became Amun-Ra, the supreme king of the gods.

Q Why was Ra depicted differently as he traveled throughout his day?

A Ra's story was a daily cycle of life and death. In the mornings, Ra journeyed across the sky in a burning boat. He was depicted as Khepri, the scarab beetle. At midday he appeared as himself because he was at the height of his power. At sunset, Ra was an old man who was swallowed by Nut, the goddess of the sky.

Q What happened to Ra after sunset?

A Ra died and sailed across the underworld. After defeating the serpent Apep, Ra was reborn to begin his journey over again.

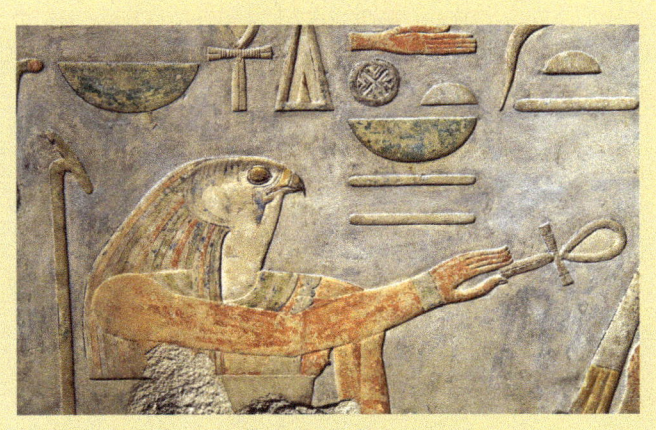

The sun god Ra reigns over Egypt.

RA'S FAMILY TREE

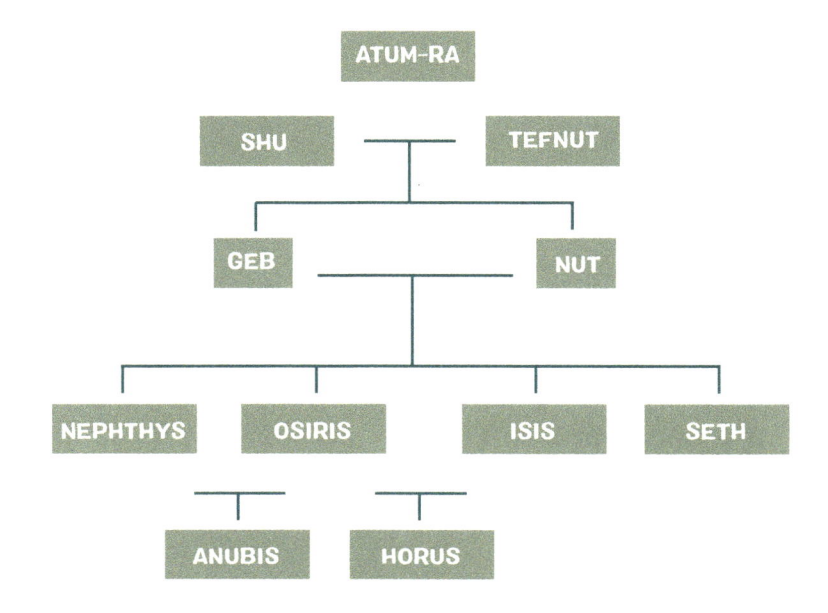

```
                    ATUM-RA
                       │
         ┌─────────────┴─────────────┐
        SHU                        TEFNUT
                       │
         ┌─────────────┴─────────────┐
        GEB                          NUT
         │
  ┌──────┬──────────┬──────────┐
NEPHTHYS OSIRIS    ISIS       SETH
            │        │
         ANUBIS   HORUS
```

Stat: There were more than 2,000 Egyptian gods and goddesses!

Q Why do some Egyptian gods have two names?

A Ancient Egypt lasted for thousands of years. Its people changed and so did their religion. Some gods rose in power only to fade in popularity later. Egyptians often combined their gods to reflect those changes.

Did You Know?

Egyptian cities often picked a main god to worship. Thebes chose Amun before he became a chief god. Memphis chose Ptah, the god of craftspeople.

TRUE OR FALSE?

The mother of all gods was named Isis.

SOMEWHAT TRUE.

Isis is the Greek name for the Egyptian goddess Aset. She was the mother of Horus and very powerful. The people worshipped her both as a protector and healer.

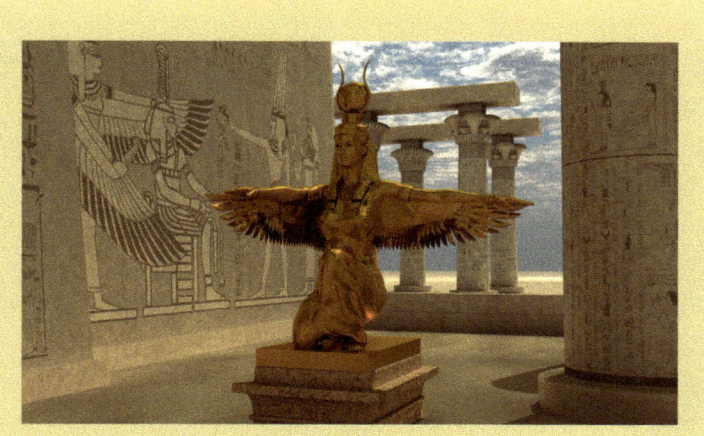

A statue of Isis, also known as Aset

RELIGIOUS ROLES 49

Did You Know?

According to Egyptian mythology, Osiris was the first king to rule the Earth. And he was doing a fine job until his brother murdered him in a fit of jealousy.

> **Stat:** Osiris's brother Seth was said to have torn Osiris into 42 pieces. He scattered the parts across the land, creating the 42 provinces of Egypt.

Q: What happened to Osiris after he was murdered?

A: After Osiris's murder, his wife, Isis, tried desperately to find all the pieces of her husband. She wanted to bring him back to life, but one piece remained hidden when it was swallowed by a fish. Isis eventually reassembled Osiris, but he was not whole. He traveled to the underworld where he became the judge of the deceased.

Q: Why is Osiris blue?

A: Blue is the color of the dead. Osiris is often depicted as a blue mummy holding the crook and flail of kingship.

Did You Know?

Egyptians believed that Horus, the son of Osiris and Isis, lived among the people as the most powerful person in Egypt: the pharaoh.

Q What happened when a pharaoh died?

A Egyptians believed that once a pharaoh entered the afterlife, they became Osiris. Their successor became the new Horus.

Q Was Anubis a werewolf?

A Nope, but Anubis is often depicted with the head of a jackal. Jackals lurked around tombs hoping to chomp on rotting flesh. These doglike animals became associated with death. Since Anubis was the god of death, mummification, and the afterlife, he was shown as half jackal.

TRUE OR FALSE?

Souls automatically continued their journey into the afterlife.

FALSE.

When a soul left its body, Anubis guided it to the Hall of Truth. Some scholars believe Osiris was the final judge of the soul. Others think Anubis determined a soul's fate.

Q Why was Anubis pictured with a balance and a feather?

A Anubis weighed the heart of the recently departed against the Feather of Truth. If the heart was balanced with the feather, the soul traveled into paradise. But if the heart was heavier, the monster Ammit ate the soul, destroying it forever.

Stat: According to Egyptian mythology, 42 judges waited for Anubis to bring the departed before them.

Did You Know?

A life-size statue of Anubis guarded the tomb of King Tut, ready to guide the spirits of the dead and punish tomb raiders.

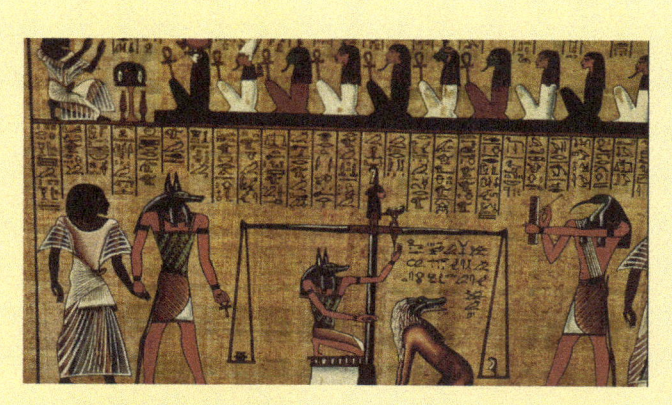

Anubis weighing the heart of the dead

Q Are those cow horns on top of Hathor's head?

A Yep. Hathor was often depicted as a heavenly cow. Her horned crown represented joy, festivity, motherhood, and beauty. She supported and celebrated dancing, music, mining, and art.

Q Was Seth an evil god?

A Stories vary about the god of chaos. In early Egyptian history, Seth granted love spells and saved Ra from an evil serpent. In later myths, Seth was sinister. He became a murderer, ruler of the unpredictable deserts, and the god of war. In animal form, he took on features of hippopotamuses or crocodiles.

Myth:
Ra was the father of all the gods.

Truth:
Thoth, the god of wisdom and the moon, was no one's child. Egyptian mythology says he emerged from the waters of Nun. Basically, he created himself. Three gods materialized with him: Khnum, Ma'at, and Ptah.

Did You Know?

Some Egyptians believed that Khnum, the ram-headed god, created humanity using his potter's wheel.

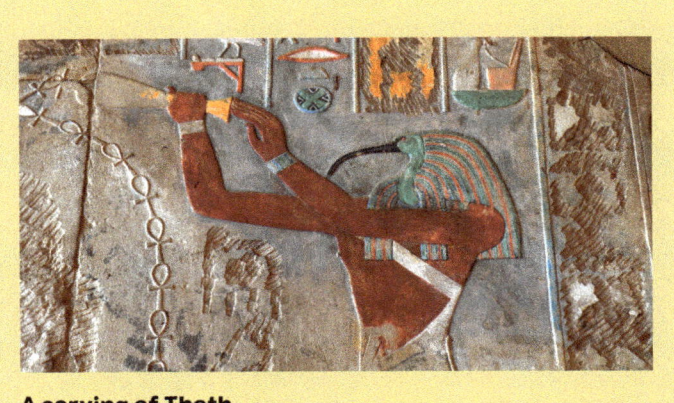

A carving of Thoth

Did You Know?

Thoth is considered the inventor of hieroglyphics. He also acted as the scribe who documented the deeds of the dead.

TIMES WHEN THOTH'S QUICK THINKING SAVED THE DAY

- **Thoth saved** Ra from the serpent on his daily journey.
- **He knew** the spell to bring Osiris back to life.
- **Thoth traded** five days' worth of moonlight for five days of sunlight so Nut could give birth to her children.

THE AFTERLIFE

Q What did ancient Egyptians believe happened after death?

A Ancient Egyptians believed death was only a beginning. They thought that the afterlife was a continuation of life on this Earth, and that Duat, the underworld, was a mirror of our world.

Q Was there a cheat sheet that helped Egyptians know how to navigate the afterlife?

A Scribes created a collection of spells to help on the journey to the afterlife. The texts are known as the Book of the Dead. It revealed ways to travel around Duat, sweet-talk the gods, and beat bad beasts.

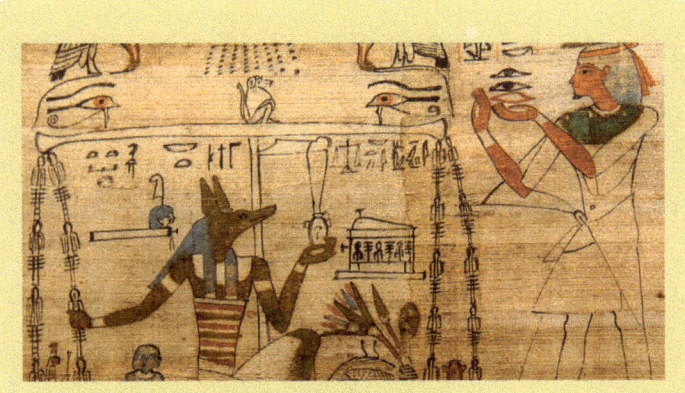

A page from the Book of the Dead

TRUE OR FALSE?

The Field of Reeds, the afterlife's paradise, was hard to reach.

TRUE.

The boat ride to the afterlife could be fraught with aggressive crocodiles, wicked spells, and other perils.

Q Why was it so important to prevent a person's body from decaying?

A According to Egyptian beliefs, people had a life force called *ka*. They also had a soul called *ba*. In order to live in the afterlife, a person needed both *ka* and *ba*. To be able to balance both these things, their bodies had to be **preserved** through the mummification process.

Q What exactly is a mummy?

A Mummies were animals or people who had perished. Their bodies were then preserved for the afterlife. Anyone *could* be made into a mummy, but only the wealthy could afford it.

Did You Know?

Embalmers, priests who made mummies, tossed out the brain during mummification. They thought it was no longer needed.

Q Why were the mummy's other organs placed in jars?

A Internal organs, like the stomach, contain water and bacteria. If they were left inside the dead, the body would rot. So, embalmers scooped the organs into vessels called "canopic jars." These jars were placed in the tomb with the mummy, where the four sons of Horus watched over them.

THE SONS OF HORUS AND THEIR CANOPIC JARS

ORGAN	PROTECTED BY	FORM ON THE LID OF THE JAR
liver	Imsety	human head
lungs	Hapy	baboon head
intestines	Qebehseneuf	falcon head
stomach	Duamutef	jackal

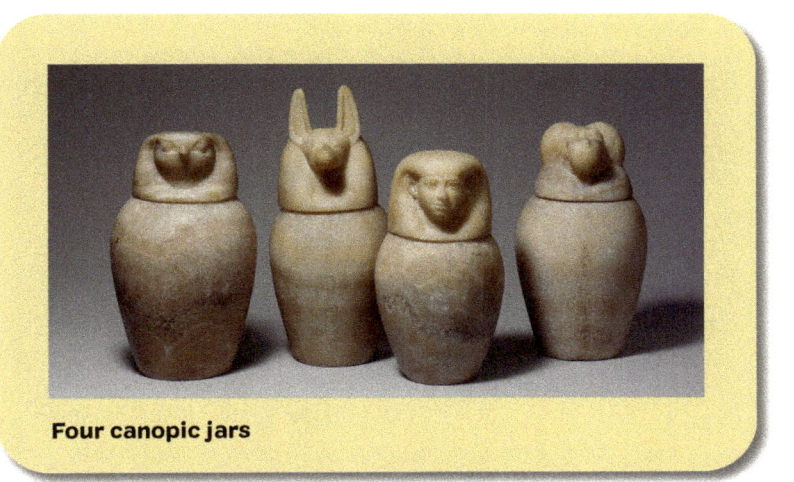

Four canopic jars

THE AFTERLIFE

Stat: It took nearly 4,000 square feet of linen to wrap one mummy. The material was stripped into bandages. The total length of the strips was about the same distance as 10 buses lined up.

Stat: It took about 70 days to mummify a body.

RECIPE FOR MAKING A MUMMY

1. Gather one corpse.
2. Wash and purify the body.
3. Hook the brain and pull it out through the nose. Throw it away.
4. Remove the lungs, liver, intestines, and stomach. Place each inside a canopic jar.
5. Be certain to leave the heart. It's the most important organ and won't be removed.
6. Pack the body with **natron**. This sucks up all the moisture.
7. Wait 40 days, then remove the natron.
8. Fill the body with rags, spices, and herbs.
9. Wrap the body tightly in several layers of linens.
10. Tuck magical **amulets** into the wrappings. Activate their protection by saying spells.
11. Place the body in a **sarcophagus**, then put it in the tomb with the jars.

Myth:
All mummies were buried in golden coffins.

Truth:
Pharaohs and royalty might have been buried in this expensive material, but most sarcophagi were made from wood or stone. Many things were carved into the surface, such as the name of the dead, food items, and a door to the afterlife.

Myth:
Tombs were filled with gold and other treasures.

Truth:
Mummies were buried with items that would be helpful during the difficult passage to the afterlife. Pharaohs had graves filled with treasures, but ordinary folk had only the basics: cosmetics, clothes, and food. These items were called "grave goods."

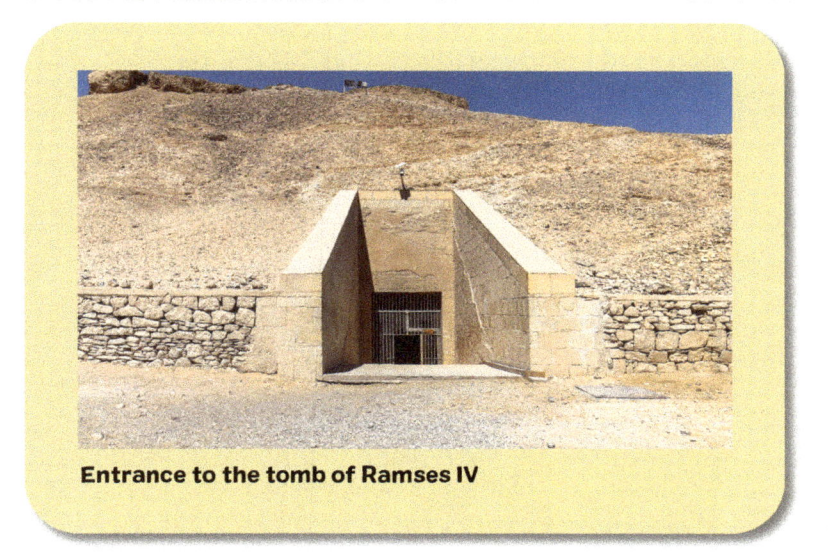

Entrance to the tomb of Ramses IV

Did You Know?

Only the rich had tombs for the afterlife.
The poor were buried in the sand.

Q Did souls go into the afterlife alone?

A Egyptians, especially wealthy ones, ventured into the afterlife with as many companions as possible. Wives, servants, and pets were buried alongside the deceased. **Shabtis** were also placed inside the tombs of the wealthy. These mini statues came to life and performed laborious tasks in place of the dead.

PACKING LIST FOR THE AFTERLIFE FOR THE RICH AND FAMOUS

clothing	elegant outfits, sandals
food	fancy breads, fruit, and meats
transportation	boats or chariots
jewelry	necklaces, elaborate headdresses, amulets for protection
other	canopic jars, shabtis, furniture, board games

Did You Know?

King Tut's tomb was filled with "meat mummies." The pharaoh couldn't go hungry in the afterlife, so even meats were mummified to give him delicacies to eat.

Q When archaeologists explored the Step Pyramid, how many mummies were found inside?

A None. Sadly, tomb robbers had stolen all of the mummified remains.

Q Why did the pharaohs have pyramids built?

A Pyramids were giant stone tombs built to last forever. Before pyramids, kings were buried in mounds of mud.

Did You Know?

After Djoser had the Step Pyramid built as his tomb, the pharaoh Sneferu took the idea and made it grander. Or at least he tried to—the first two attempts failed! The third try, the Red Pyramid, still stands today.

FOUR FAMOUS PYRAMIDS

PYRAMID	HEIGHT	BUILT FOR	LOCATION
The Great Pyramid	455 feet (139 meters)	Khufu	Giza
Pyramid of Khafre	448 feet (136.5 meters)	Khafre	Giza
Red Pyramid	341 feet (104 meters)	Sneferu	Dashur
Step Pyramid	200 feet (61 meters)	Djoser	Saqqara

Did You Know?

The Red Pyramid was considered the first "true pyramid." True pyramids have smooth sides. The sides of King Djoser's stony tomb were like stairs.

TRUE OR FALSE?

More than 130 pyramids have been discovered in the sands of Egyptian dunes.

TRUE.

Experts believe that even more pyramids may be hidden in the desert, but only time will tell.

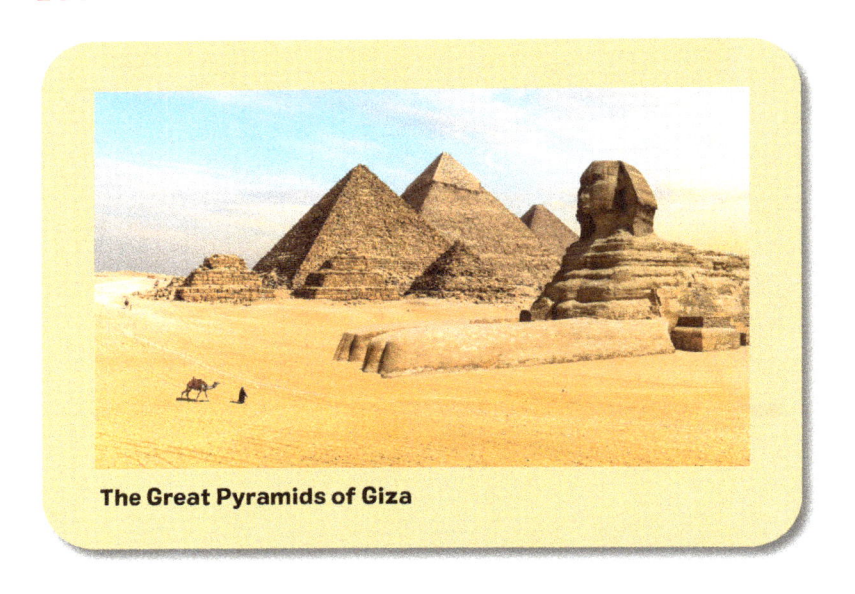

The Great Pyramids of Giza

Stat: Some stones used to build the pyramids weighed more than an elephant! In fact, some weighed more than 70 tons, or around 10 elephants.

Q Besides pyramids, tombs, and temples, what other types of monuments did pharaohs build?

A Giant statues like the Great Sphinx at Giza were created for pharaohs. The Colossi of Memnon, which portrayed the pharaoh Amenhotep III, stood at 60 feet tall.

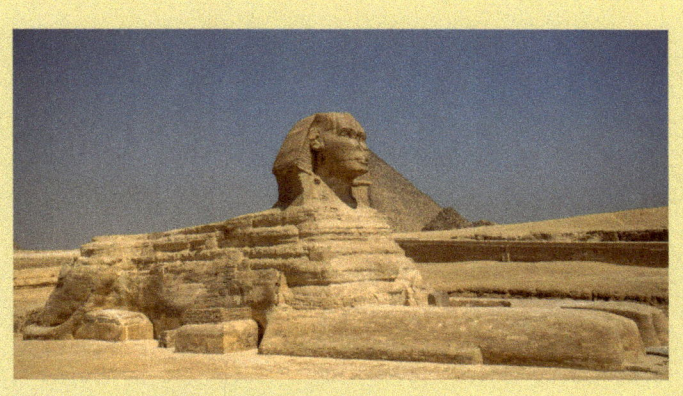

The Great Sphinx at Giza

THE DIRT ON SPHINXES

Sphinxes are mythological creatures.

Their role is to guard tombs and temples.

The Great Sphinx at Giza is around 241 feet (73.5 meters) long. It stands at 66 feet (20 meters) high!

There are three kinds of sphinx. *Androsphinx* has the body of a lion and the head of a person. *Criosphinx* has the body of a lion and the head of a ram. *Hieracosphinx* has the body of a lion and the head of a hawk.

At one point in its history, the Great Sphinx had a beard.

Did You Know?

In both Egyptian and Greek mythology, the Great Sphinx terrorized the city of Thebes (also called Luxor) by killing all those who could not solve its riddle.

Q What happened to the nose of the Great Sphinx at Giza?

A No one knows for sure. Some say it broke because of weathering and erosion from sand and wind.

Stat: About 1,350 sphinxes line the road between the temples at Karnak and Luxor. Called the Avenue of Sphinxes, its construction began during the Middle Kingdom.

TALES FROM THE TOMBS

Q Were pyramids totally open on the inside?

A No. What you see is pretty much what you get when it comes to Egyptian pyramids. Many stones were stacked to create the shape of the pyramid. That design left little space for anything but a few **chambers**.

Q How many rooms were in a pyramid?

A There were three main **chambers** in tombs. Below the surface was the burial chamber where the sarcophagus rested with its canopic jars and afterlife treasures. Above ground, there was the Queen's Chamber and a long hall called the Grand Gallery.

Myth:
Queens were buried in the Queen's Chamber of the Great Pyramid of Giza.

Truth:
The chamber was misnamed by archaeologists who were exploring Khufu's tomb.

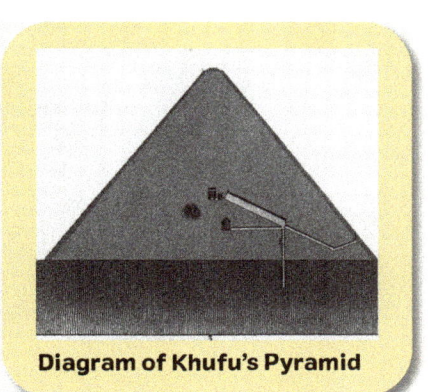

Diagram of Khufu's Pyramid

Did You Know?

After the Middle Kingdom, pharaohs no longer built pyramids. Instead, they were buried in tombs carved into the walls of a dried-up riverbed called the Valley of the Kings. Many famous pharaohs' tombs are located in the valley, including those of Thutmose II, Ramses II, Hatshepsut, and King Tut.

Q: Why did the pharaohs choose to be buried in the Valley of the Kings?

A: Scholars aren't certain why. Many historians think the pharaohs moved their burial ground to the valley to avoid their tombs being raided.

Did You Know?

A **necropolis** is a large and elaborate burial place often built with stone monuments. Necropolis comes from a Greek word meaning "city of the dead."

Myth:
The only necropolis is the Valley of the Kings.

Truth:
There are many necropolises, like the Valley of the Queens, the Valley of the Nobles, and even a necropolis for pets!

TRUE OR FALSE?

Egyptians painted or carved false doors on tomb walls.

TRUE.

Fake doors were common temple decorations. These doors were thought to be portals that allowed the dead or even the gods to enter the living world.

Did You Know?

No one entered a tomb once it was sealed. Instead, people left food and gifts in front of the false doors for their departed family.

Did You Know?

King Tut's tomb had been **looted** at least twice before its discovery, but it's still one of the most intact tombs ever found. Archaeologists learned much about ancient Egypt because of it!

Stat: Tutankhamun's sarcophagus was made entirely out of gold and weighed more than 200 pounds.

Stat: The treasures inside King Tut's tomb were rumored to be worth $750 million. Tutankhamun's coffin is estimated to cost $13 million alone!

Myth:
Hieroglyphics were the only writings inscribed on the walls of tombs.

Truth:
Egyptians decorated tombs with bright pictures celebrating their families and memorable life events. Tomb walls also had curses for would-be tomb raiders.

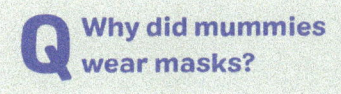

Q Why did mummies wear masks?

A Egyptians wanted the soul of the deceased to recognize and return to its body. The masks had bright open eyes and huge smiles. Most masks were made of wood or cartonnage, a mix of papyrus and cloth soaked in plaster. Royal masks were crafted with precious metals like gold or bronze.

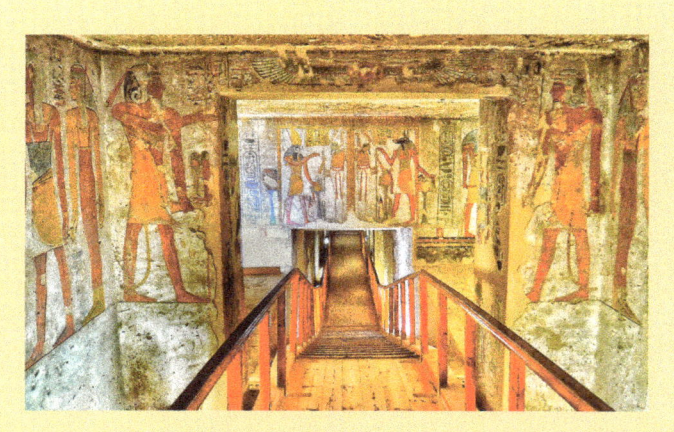

Hieroglyphics line the walls inside the Valley of the Kings.

Q What is the curse of the pharaohs?

A A curse is rumored to befall anyone who disturbs the eternal rest of a mummy.

Q Is King Tut's curse real?

A It's debatable. The rumor started after the archaeologist Howard Carter and his team entered King Tut's tomb in 1922 CE. Shortly after, bad things started happening to the crew. First, Carter's pet canary was eaten by a cobra. Next, Carter's boss, Lord Carnavon, died from a mosquito bite. Finally, Carter's friend, who helped him with the dig, had his house burn down. Twice.

Myth:
Ancient Egyptians built deadly traps for would-be thieves.

Truth:
Egyptians went to great lengths to deter tomb raiders. They built false walls and large pits, and they sealed off chambers with plaster doors. They carved warnings and curses into the tomb walls. They even hid the chambers behind boulders and rubble. But they did not booby-trap the tombs with sharp stakes or crush raiders with rolling rocks. That happens only in action scenes in movies!

Q Why was the village of Deir el-Medina built outside the Valley of the Kings?

A The purpose of the city and its citizens was to prevent tomb robberies. It worked for a while. But when supplies grew scarce, some villagers resorted to doing exactly what they were trying to stop: burial chamber burglary!

Q Where have all the mummies gone?

A Sadly, mummies were not left in their final resting places for many reasons. Thieves burned them to melt down golden treasures. Mummies were sold for parts. And around the year 1800 CE, Europeans experienced "Egyptomania," a fad for all things Egyptian. They stole souvenirs from their trips to Egypt, including mummies.

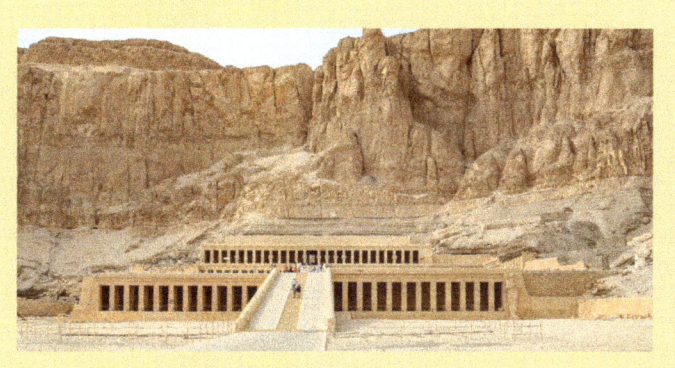

Outside the Valley of the Kings

WHAT WERE MUMMIES USED FOR DURING EGYPTOMANIA?

- fertilizers
- household decorations
- medicine
- paint
- party entertainment
- stage props

TRUE OR FALSE?

Europeans held mummy-unwrapping parties.

TRUE.

During the 1830s, it became common for European nobles to hold parties where a mummy was unwrapped. More than 2,000 people paid to attend Thomas Pettigrew's public unwrapping of a mummy in London.

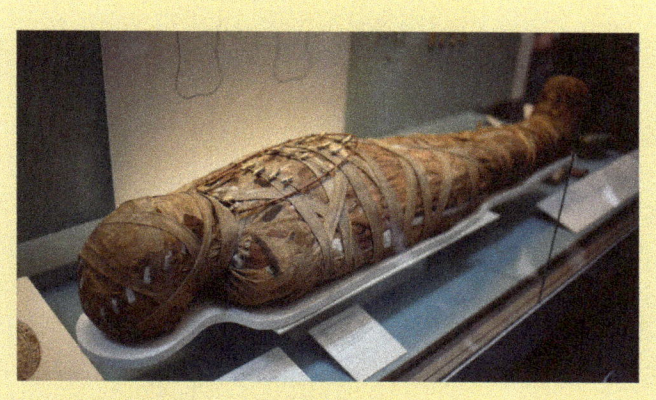

A mummy in a modern museum

TALES FROM THE TOMBS

Myth:
The *Titanic* sank because an Egyptian mummy was on board.

Truth:
The ship's manifest, or supply list, had no record of a mummy setting sail with the doomed vessel.

Q Is it illegal to take a mummy out of Egypt?

A Yes. Egypt has passed many laws protecting their mummies. Over time, many countries around the world have sought to return the dead and their treasures. Theft of the ancient artifacts is still a problem today.

Did You Know?

One mummy has received permission to travel. Ramses II has his own passport, which he used to visit France in 1974.

Q Where can tourists go see mummies today?

A Mummies can be seen in museums around the world. In 2021, 22 royal mummies were moved to the National Museum of Egyptian Civilization in Egypt, including Ramses II, Thutmose II, and Hatshepsut.

THE UPS AND DOWNS OF EGYPT

Q Why was Ramses III considered the last of the great pharaohs?

A Like pharaohs before him, Ramses III sought to expand **foreign** trade. He built monuments, reorganized the government, and built temples. He even started a tree-planting program. His efforts, however, were not well received. His wife tried to overthrow and murder him. Egypt's power and prominence began to dwindle after his reign.

THE END OF ANCIENT EGYPT

1213 BCE	Ramses III dies.
1100 BCE	Egypt splits into two kingdoms during a civil war.
730 to 305 BCE	Egypt faces foreign invasion from Nubia, Assyria, and Persia.
305 BCE	Ptolemy gains control of Egypt, establishing the last dynasty.
30 BCE	Cleopatra, the last pharaoh, dies. This ends the pharaonic period.

Myth:
Ancient Egyptians are known only for building pyramids.

Truth:
Ancient Egyptians invented or adapted many innovations that we still use today, including paper, ink, locks, and more!

Did You Know?

Egyptians created the first police force. They even used animals like dogs and monkeys to help catch criminals.

Did You Know?

Ancient Egyptians did not use vowels in their written language. What would Old MacDonald have done?!

Q Were hieroglyphics the only form of writing in ancient Egypt?

A No. After hieroglyphics, Egyptians developed two other styles of writing. Hieratic was mainly used by priests. The second form was called "demotic." It was used more by the common people. When Napoleon conquered Egypt, his team discovered the Rosetta Stone. This stone tablet contained text in all three styles.

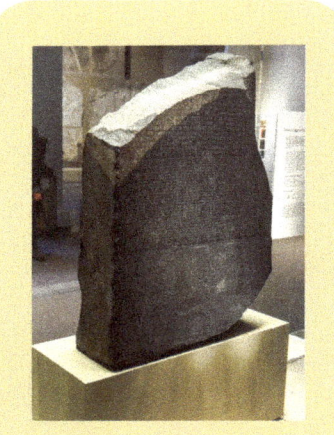

The Rosetta Stone on display at a museum

Myth:
Egyptians carved *everything* into stone tablets, walls, and sarcophagi.

Truth:
Egyptians invented paper. The process for making these sheets from river plants was a closely guarded secret!

Q Did Egyptians invent libraries, too?

A No. However, Egyptians had one of the largest and most important libraries in the ancient world! The Great Library of Alexandria was open to royals and ordinary citizens alike, but no one could take its papyrus scrolls home to read. The Great Library was rumored to have more than 500,000 scrolls, organized in genres such as tragic poetry, comedy, medicine, and law. This "house of books" was later destroyed during an invasion and its treasures were lost.

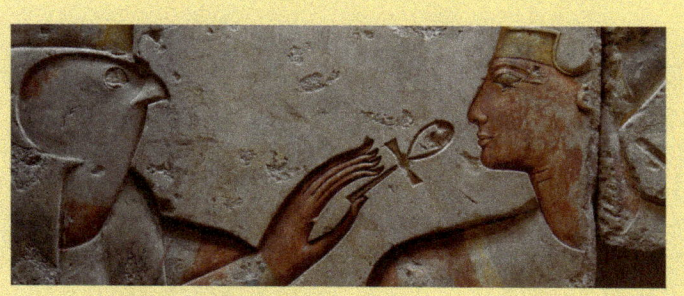

Horus blesses the Pharaoh

Q What exactly was a "house" in ancient Egypt?

A Egyptians called important places "houses," but they didn't live in them. For example, tombs were "houses of eternity." Libraries were "houses of books." "Houses of life" were educational centers where priests and scribes studied reading, writing, medicine, geography, dream interpretation, mathematics, and more. Houses of life were also where copies of the Book of the Dead were made.

Did You Know?

Egyptians invented the first clocks. Giant **obelisks** cast shadows onto engravings to mark time, much like sundials. Egyptians also used water clocks that dripped as time passed.

Did You Know?

Ancient Egyptians were the first people to use a calendar with 365 days.

Myth:
Americans invented bowling.

Truth:
It was the Egyptians! One of the earliest games of bowling was discovered during an excavation of a tomb that dated back to 5200 BCE. Corn husks and string balls were launched at pins made from stone.

Did You Know?

Ghastly ghosts, demons, and evil spirits were believed to cause illnesses and diseases. That didn't stop Egyptians from developing effective medicines and health practices.

Q: Who helped the sick in ancient Egypt?

A: Because magic and medicine were one and the same, priests were often doctors as well. They cast spells, prescribed amulets, and whipped up remedies. Some of their medicine might seem strange to us today, like boiled mice to cure coughs and crocodile poop for aches and bruises.

Did You Know?

Egyptians were the first barbers. Because of heat and lice, Egyptian men and women often shaved their heads.

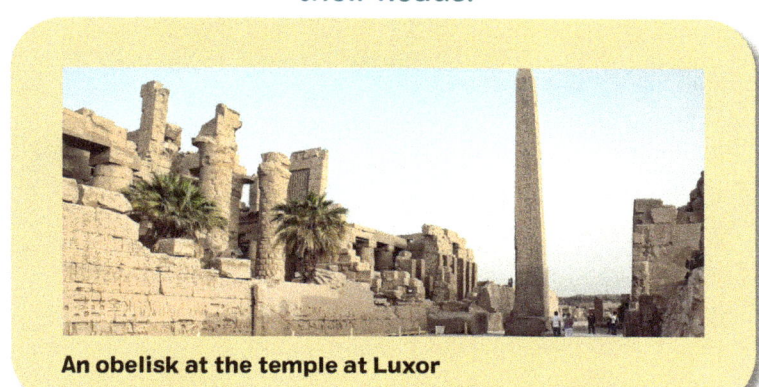

An obelisk at the temple at Luxor

Myth:
Makeup was meant only for looking good.

Truth:
Not only did cosmetics protect the wearers from the burning sun, the minerals prevented eye diseases and infections.

Q Did ancient Egyptians use antibiotics to help the sick?

A Egyptians were some of the first to develop antibiotics. But the medicines weren't like the ones we use today. In fact, they used moldy bread to fight off infections! The bread was stuffed into a wound to kill germs.

Q If staying healthy was important, how did Egyptians take care of their teeth?

A Egyptians invented toothpaste to help fight tooth decay. They used their fingers or twigs as a toothbrush.

Did You Know?

Bad breath plagued ancient Egyptians, too! Their solution? They invented the first breath mints. Boiled honey mixed with spices like cinnamon fought off nasty breath.

GLOSSARY

alliance: A friendship or relationship between two groups of people to accomplish a goal

amulet: A small token that protects against evil and danger

archaeologist: A person who studies history by digging for objects from the past

barter: To trade one thing for another; no money is exchanged, only items

bureaucracy: A group of people who work for the government

chamber: A room in a tomb

clergy: The workers and leaders of a religious group

deities: Gods and goddesses

dwell: To live in a place

dynasty: A line of rulers from the same family

embalmer: A person who prepares a dead body for the afterlife so that it does not decay

exile: Forcing someone to leave their country or home

foreign: From a different country

heretic: A person who believes or teaches something that goes against a particular religion

loot: To steal or take by force

natron: Salt used to remove moisture

necropolis: A large cemetery near an ancient city

nomad: A person who has no permanent home but moves from place to place

obelisk: A stone pillar

phenomenon: An observable event in nature

polytheistic: Believing in many gods

preserve: To keep safe from ruin or decay

regent: A person who rules in place of a monarch who is too young or unable to lead

sarcophagus: A large box used to bury the dead

shabti: A small statue buried in Egyptian tombs; these figurines were thought to come alive and serve the deceased

succession: One person following after another

supreme: The highest in rank

tomb: A grave or burial place

vizier: The second in command to the ruler, who offers advice and helps rule the kingdom

RESOURCES

Want to find out more about ancient Egypt? Start here! Use Google Maps, Smithsonian Journeys, or YouTube 360° to take a virtual field trip.

VIRTUAL TOURS
Abu Simbel
Luxor Temple
The Pyramids of Giza
The Temple of Karnak

WEBSITES
DK Find Out!
DKFindOut.com/us/history/ancient-egypt

History for Kids
HistoryForKids.net/ancient-egypt.html

National Geographic for Kids: Ancient Egypt
NatGeoKids.com/ie/tag/ancient-egypt

BOOKS
Hart, George. *Eyewitness: Ancient Egypt.* London: DK Children, 2014.

Morley, Jacqueline. *You Wouldn't Want to Be a Pyramid Builder!* Brighton, UK: Book House, 2018.

ACKNOWLEDGMENTS

Any sort of research takes long hours, many eyes, and many hands. A huge thank you to my wonderful editor, Eliza, who answered a million questions and made this project possible. And a colossal shout-out to my husband and bestie, who learned more about Egypt than they ever thought possible.

ABOUT THE AUTHOR

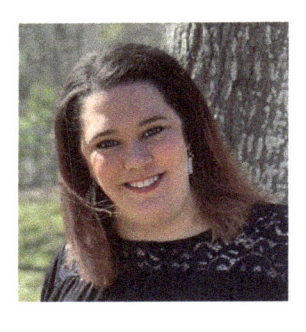

Combine humor and a love of picture books. Stir in noisy kids and a handsome husband. Add a pinch of teaching, a dash of being a librarian, and *voilà*! You have the author **Ciara O'Neal**. This busy mom loves reading, silly puns, and underwater basket weaving. She plots world domination with a donut in each hand.